JUICING FOR DIABETES REVERSAL

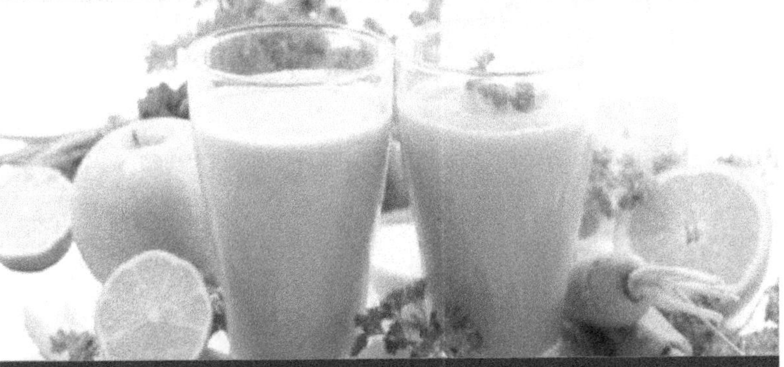

Quick, Easy Recipes To Manage And Reverse Type 1 And Type 2 Diabetes

LEONA BUTLER

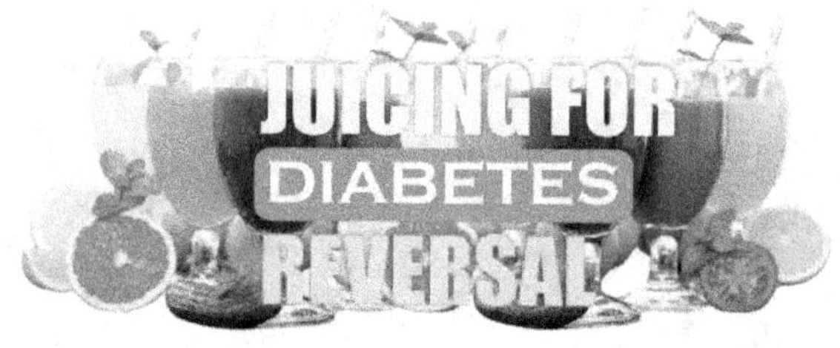
JUICING FOR
DIABETES
REVERSAL

TABLE OF CONTENT

Introduction

Larry, a tough old man, had been battling diabetes for years. He discovered the magic of juicing after becoming dissatisfied with standard treatments. Intriguingly, he began a daily regimen of freshly squeezed fruits and vegetables.

Larry gradually noticed improvements in his health.
His concoction contained antioxidant-rich kale, spinach, and berries, all of which were intended to stabilize blood sugar levels. The brilliant colors represented his internal metamorphosis. Larry's perseverance paid off; his diabetes was being reversed.

Larry's incredible trip became known throughout the neighborhood. Neighbors sought his guidance, and a juicing community sprang up. Larry rose to the status of neighborhood health guru, combining wisdom and produce to inspire others.

Larry's vigor shifted with the seasons. His zest for life returned as he thrived on the nutrients in his homemade juices. Larry's story reverberated far beyond his little town, giving hope to those facing similar health issues. Larry discovered not only a treatment but also a purpose in the rhythm of juicing: to share the gift of wellness with a world yearning for solutions.

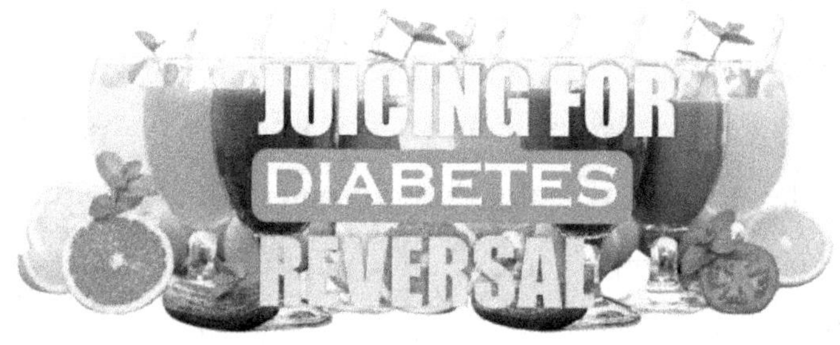

The diabetes, types, it's cause, symptoms and preventive measures.

Diabetes is a chronic metabolic disorder characterized by elevated levels of blood glucose, resulting from either insufficient insulin production or the body's inability to effectively use insulin.

There are primarily two types of diabetes: Type 1 and Type 2.

Type 1 Diabetes

Type 1 diabetes is an autoimmune disease in which the immune system assaults and destroys insulin-producing beta cells in the pancreas by mistake. This causes a lack of insulin, a hormone essential for controlling blood sugar levels. This kind typically manifests in childhood or adolescence and necessitates lifetime insulin therapy. Type 1 diabetes is caused by a combination of genetic and environmental factors.

Type 2 Diabetes

Type 2 diabetes is more common and is frequently connected with lifestyle factors. The body develops resistant to insulin in this state, and the pancreas may not generate enough insulin to meet the increasing demand. Obesity, sedentary living, heredity, and age are all significant risk factors for Type 2 diabetes. Because of increased obesity rates, it is increasingly being diagnosed in children and adolescents.

Common Symptoms

Excessive thirst, frequent urination, unexplained weight loss, exhaustion, and blurred vision are all symptoms shared by both forms of diabetes. Because of changing blood sugar levels, people with Type 1 diabetes may experience irritation and mood changes. These symptoms are caused by the body's inability to adequately utilize glucose, resulting in increased quantities in the bloodstream.

Causes

Diabetes Type 1 and Type 2 have different causes. Type 1 diabetes is caused mostly by genetic factors as well as an autoimmune response that attacks insulin-producing cells. Triggers in the environment, such as viral infections, may also play a role. Type 2 diabetes, on the other hand, is closely connected to lifestyle variables such as poor diet, lack of physical activity, and obesity. Although genetic predisposition can enhance the risk, lifestyle decisions also play an important part in its development.

Preventive Measures

Healthy Lifestyle: Adopting a healthy lifestyle is critical for Type 2 diabetes prevention. Part of this includes eating a balanced diet rich in fruits, vegetables, whole grains, and lean meats. Physical activity on a regular basis helps with weight control and insulin sensitivity.

Weight Control: Maintaining a healthy weight is critical in the prevention and management of Type 2 diabetes. Obesity is a key risk factor, and even modest weight loss can have a big impact on insulin resistance reduction.

Regular Physical Activity: Being physically active on a regular basis helps regulate blood sugar levels, increases insulin sensitivity, and promotes overall cardiovascular health. Aim for at least 150 minutes of moderate-intensity exercise every week.

Balanced Diet: Choose a diet that is rich in complex carbohydrates, healthy fats, and lean proteins. Reduce your consumption of refined sugars and processed meals. Portion control is critical for weight management.

Routine Health Check-ups: Regular health check-ups and screenings are critical for the early detection and management of diabetes. Monitoring blood sugar, blood pressure, and cholesterol levels can assist in identifying potential problems before they become serious.

Avoid Smoking and Limit Alcohol use: Smoking raises the risk of diabetes complications, while excessive alcohol use can cause blood sugar levels to fluctuate. Quitting smoking and limiting alcohol consumption improve general health.

The juice to drink or avoid on a diabetes to achieve optimum health.

Choosing the proper beverages is critical to maintaining optimal diabetes health. Because the effect of juices on blood sugar levels vary it is critical to be selective in beverage choices. While some juices can be part of a healthy diabetes diet, others should be drunk in moderation or avoided entirely.

To begin, it is critical to recognize that whole fruits are often preferred over fruit liquids. Whole fruits contain fiber, which slows sugar absorption and aids with blood sugar regulation. When fruits are juiced, however, their fiber content is often reduced or eliminated. A lack of fiber can cause blood sugar levels to climb more quickly.

Vegetable juices are frequently recommended as juices that can be included in a diabetes-friendly diet. These juices, especially those containing low-carbohydrate vegetables such as spinach, kale, and cucumber, can supply critical nutrients without generating large blood sugar rises. Adding lemon or lime juice to water can also add taste without significantly increasing the sugar content.

Many commercial fruit juices, on the other hand, have added sugars and high levels of natural sugars, making them unsuitable for diabetics. These liquids can cause fast rises in blood sugar levels, complicating glucose management. It's best to read nutrition labels and choose 100% fruit juices with no added sugars, but even then, moderation is crucial.

Orange juice is one juice to be wary of. Despite its popularity as a breakfast option, its high sugar content can cause a rapid rise in blood sugar. This impact can be mitigated by using a smaller serving size or diluting it with water. Furthermore, choosing whole oranges versus orange juice includes fiber, which helps regulate sugar absorption.

Sugary beverages, such as sodas and energy drinks, should be avoided because they might have a negative impact on blood sugar levels. These beverages frequently include high fructose corn syrup and provide empty calories, which contribute to weight gain and insulin resistance.

Individuals with diabetes should drink water as their primary beverage. Water has no effect on blood sugar levels, therefore staying hydrated is essential for overall health. Herbal teas with no added sugars can be enjoyed as well, giving flavor without the hazards associated with sugary beverages.

The core benefits of following Juicing for diabetes reversal for beginners (or seniors).

Juicing delivers a concentrated amount of key nutrients from fruits and vegetables, which benefits general health. Focus on low-glycemic foods like leafy greens, berries, and cucumbers for diabetes reversal.

Blood Sugar Control: Certain juices, such as green vegetable blends, may aid in blood sugar regulation by supplying nutrients that promote insulin sensitivity.

Staying hydrated is essential for diabetic management. Juicing provides a tasty approach to drink more fluids, hence ensuring optimal hydration.

Weight Loss: Including fresh juices in your diet will help you lose weight, which is important in diabetes treatment. To improve satiety, choose fiber-rich foods.

Fruits and vegetables are high in antioxidants, which help to fight oxidative stress. This has the potential to help prevent diabetes complications.

Improved Digestion: By supplying enzymes and fiber, juices can assist digestion. To support gastrointestinal health, choose high-fiber fruits and vegetables such as apple or pear.

Detoxification: Certain vegetables, such as beets and leafy greens, may help the body's natural detoxification processes, potentially improving general health.

Juicing provides an easy approach to ingest a range of nutrients in one glass, which is especially beneficial for those who have difficulty chewing or digesting entire fruits and vegetables.

Before making significant dietary changes, remember to speak with a healthcare expert, especially if you have a pre-existing health issue like diabetes.

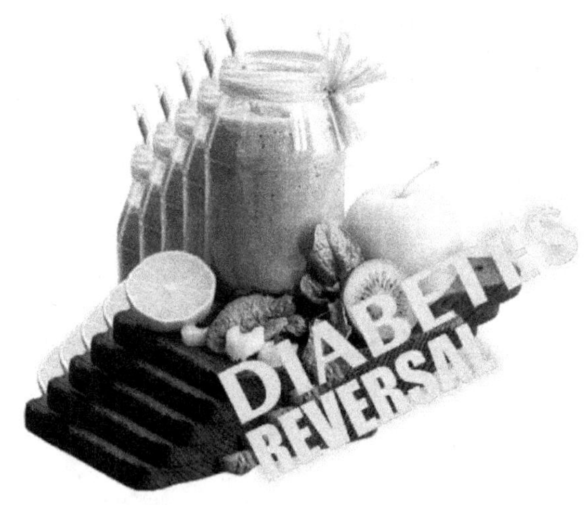

The complications of Juicing for diabetes reversals if the right diet isn't adopted.

While juicing can be a healthy part of some people's diets, including those with diabetes, it's important to be aware of potential problems. Inappropriate juicing techniques may result in:

Increased Sugar Intake: Fruits, which contain natural sugars, are frequently utilized in juices. Large amounts of fruit juice can induce a quick jump in blood sugar levels, which can be dangerous for diabetics.

Juicing frequently removes the fiber contained in whole fruits and vegetables. Fiber aids in blood sugar regulation and intestinal wellness. There is a possibility of faster sugar absorption if it is not present.

Calorie Overconsumption: Juices can be calorie-dense, and excessive calorie intake may contribute to weight gain, thereby exacerbating insulin resistance in diabetics.

Imbalance in critical Nutrients: Relying entirely on juices may result in an imbalance in critical nutrients such as proteins and healthy fats, all of which are essential for overall health and diabetic management.

troubles with water: Some juicing programs may not give proper water, which is critical for diabetics to help prevent complications such as kidney troubles.

Individual Blood Sugar Response Variability: Individual responses to juices can differ. It is critical to regularly monitor your blood sugar levels and understand how different drinks influence you.

Before introducing juicing into a diabetes treatment strategy, contact with a healthcare professional or a qualified dietitian to avoid these issues. They can assist you in developing a balanced and personalized approach that is tailored to your specific health requirements.

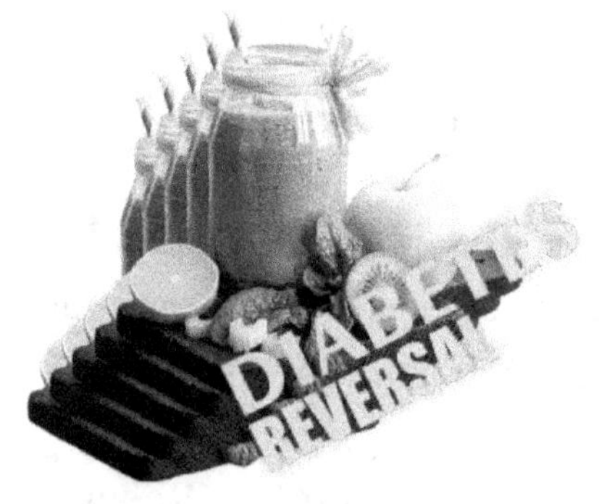

1. Green juices for diabetes reversal

1. Kale and cucumber delight

Ingredients

2 cups fresh kale, chopped

large cucumber, thinly sliced

1/4 cup cherry tomatoes, halved

1/4 cup red onion, finely diced

1/4 cup feta cheese, crumbled

tablespoons extra virgin olive oil

1 tablespoon balsamic vinegar Salt and pepper to taste

Preparation:

1. In a large bowl, combine the chopped kale, sliced cucumber, halved cherry tomatoes, diced red onion, and crumbled feta cheese.

2. In a small bowl, whisk together the extra virgin olive oil and balsamic vinegar. Drizzle the dressing over the salad.

3. Toss the salad gently to ensure all ingredients are well coated with the dressing.

4. Season to taste with salt and pepper.

5. Allow the salad to marinate for at least 15 minutes to let the flavors meld.

Nutritional Value:

- Kale is high in A, C, and K vitamins, as well as fiber and antioxidants.
- Cucumbers provide hydration, vitamins K and C, and are low in calories.
- Tomatoes contribute vitamin C and lycopene.
- Feta cheese adds protein and calcium.

Juicy Time:

For optimal juiciness, enjoy the salad after it has marinated for at least 15 minutes. The flavors will intensify, creating a delightful and refreshing experience.

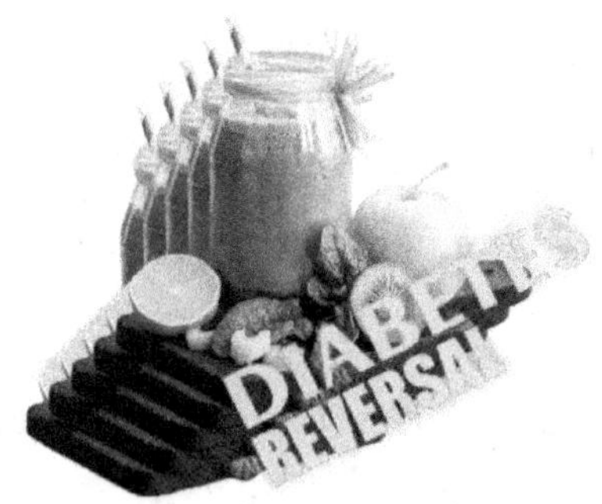

2. Spinach ginger zing

Ingredients:

2 cups cleaned and sliced fresh spinach leaves

1 tablespoon grated ginger

1 tablespoon olive oil

1 clove garlic, minced

1 teaspoon lemon zest

Salt and pepper to taste

Preparation:

1. In a skillet over medium heat, heat the olive oil.

2. Add minced garlic and grated ginger, sauté for 1-2 minutes until fragrant.

3. Add chopped spinach to the pan, stirring until wilted.

4. Sprinkle lemon zest over the spinach, mix well.

5. Season with salt and pepper to taste.

6. Cook for an additional 2-3 minutes until flavors meld. Serve immediately.

Nutritional Value (per serving):

- Calories: 80

- Protein: 4g

- Fat: 6g

- Carbohydrates: 5g

- Fiber: 2g

3. Spinach and green apple delight

Ingredients:

- 2 cups cleaned and sliced fresh spinach leaves

- 1 green apple, cored and diced

- 1/4 cup feta cheese, crumbled

- 1/4 cup walnuts, chopped

- 1 tablespoon olive oil

- 1 tablespoon balsamic vinegar Salt and pepper to taste

Preparation:

- In a large bowl, combine the fresh spinach, diced green apple, crumbled feta cheese, and chopped walnuts.
- In a small bowl, whisk together olive oil and balsamic vinegar. Drizzle the dressing over the salad.
- Gently toss the ingredients until well combined. Season with salt and pepper to taste.
- Serve immediately as a refreshing salad or side dish.

Nutritional Value (per serving):

- Calories: ~220
- Protein: ~6g
- Carbohydrates: ~15g
- Fiber: ~4g
- Fat: ~16g
- Vitamin A: ~60% DV
- Vitamin C: ~20% DV
- Calcium: ~10% DV
- Iron: ~15% DV

4. Refreshing Cucumber Spinach Cooler:

Ingredients:

- medium cucumber, peeled and sliced

- cups fresh spinach leaves

- 1 cup ice cubes

- 1/2 cup plain Greek yogurt

- 1 tablespoon fresh lemon juice

- 1 teaspoon honey (optional)

- 1/2 teaspoon grated ginger

- 1/4 teaspoon salt

- Fresh mint leaves for garnish

Preparation:

1. In a blender, combine cucumber slices, spinach leaves, ice cubes, Greek yogurt, lemon juice, honey (if using), grated ginger, and salt.

2. Blend on high speed until smooth and creamy.

3. Taste and adjust sweetness or saltiness if needed.

4. Pour the cooler into glasses and garnish with fresh mint leaves.

5. Serve immediately and enjoy this nutrient-packed, hydrating beverage!

Nutritional Value (per serving):

- Calories: Approximately 80
- Protein: 5g
- Carbohydrates: 10g
- Fiber: 2g
- Sugars: 5g
- Fat: 2g
- Vitamin C: 20% of daily recommended intake
- Vitamin A: 50% of daily recommended intake

5. Avocado kale twist

Ingredients:

- 2 ripe avocados
- 4 cups fresh kale, chopped
- lemon (juiced)
- tablespoons olive oil
- 1 garlic clove, minced
- Salt and pepper to taste
- Optional toppings: cherry tomatoes, pumpkin seeds

Preparation:

Avocado Mash:

1. Peel and pit the avocados, then mash them in a bowl.

2.   Add lemon juice to prevent browning.

3.   Season with salt and pepper.

Sautéed Kale:

1.   In a skillet over medium heat, heat the olive oil. Sauté minced garlic until fragrant.

2.   Add chopped kale and cook until wilted but still vibrant.

3.   Season with salt and pepper.

Assembly:

1.   Spread a generous layer of avocado mash on a plate.

2.   Top with sautéed kale mixture.

3.   Garnish with optional toppings like cherry tomatoes and pumpkin seeds.

Nutritional Value (per serving):

- Calories: Approximately 300

- Healthy fats from avocados

- Rich in fiber from kale

- Good source of vitamins C and K Provides essential minerals like potassium

Enjoy this nutritious Avocado Kale Twist!

6. celery spinach green juice

Ingredients:

- 2 cups fresh spinach leaves

- 1 cup chopped celery

- 1 green apple, cored and sliced

- 1 cucumber, peeled and chopped

- 1 lemon, juiced

- 1/2 inch ginger, peeled

- 1 cup cold water or coconut water Ice cubes (optional)

Preparation:

1. Wash the spinach leaves, celery, apple, and cucumber thoroughly.
2. In a blender, combine spinach, celery, green apple, cucumber, lemon juice, and ginger.
3. Add cold water or coconut water for desired consistency.
4. Blend until smooth.
5. Strain the juice using a fine mesh sieve or cheesecloth to remove pulp if desired.
6. Pour the juice into a glass over ice cubes, if preferred.

Nutritional Value:

- Calories: Approximately 120 kcal
- Protein: 3g
- Carbohydrates: 30g
- Dietary Fiber: 8g
- Fat: 1g
- Vitamins and Minerals: Rich in vitamin A, C, K, potassium, and folate.

Ingredients:

- 2 cups cleaned and sliced fresh spinach leaves
- 1 tablespoon olive oil
- teaspoon grated ginger
- cloves garlic, minced
- 1/2 teaspoon cumin seeds Salt and pepper to taste

Preparation:

1. In a skillet over medium heat, heat the olive oil.
2. Allow the cumin seeds to crackle for a few seconds.
3. Add minced garlic and grated ginger, sauté until fragrant.
4. Add chopped spinach, stirring occasionally, cook until wilted.
5. Season with salt and pepper to taste.
6. Remove from heat and serve.

Nutritional Value (per serving):

- Calories: 80

- Protein: 3g

- Fat: 6g

- Carbohydrates: 5g

- Fiber: 2g

- Vitamin A: 150% DV

- Vitamin C: 30% DV

- Iron: 15% DV

8. Brussels sprouts berry burst

Ingredients:

- 500g Brussels sprouts, halved

- cup berries (strawberries, raspberries, and blueberries)

- tablespoons olive oil

- tablespoon balsamic vinegar

- Salt and pepper to taste

- tablespoons honey

Preparation:

1. Preheat the oven to 400°F (200°C).

2. In a large mixing bowl, toss Brussels sprouts with olive oil, balsamic vinegar, salt, and pepper until evenly coated.

3. Spread the Brussels sprouts on a baking sheet in a single layer.

4. Roast in the preheated oven for 20-25 minutes or until golden brown and crispy, stirring halfway through.

5. While the Brussels sprouts are roasting, mix the mixed berries with honey in a separate bowl. Once the Brussels sprouts are done, transfer them to a serving dish and top with the berry mixture.

Nutritional Value (per serving):

- Calories: 250
- Protein: 6g
- Fat: 14g
- Carbohydrates: 30g
- Fiber: 8g
- Sugars: 15g
- Vitamin C: 90mg

- Iron: 2mg

9. Green Collard Bliss

Ingredients:

- 1 bunch of fresh green collard greens

- tablespoon olive oil

- cloves garlic, minced

- 1/2 teaspoon red pepper flakes (optional)

- Salt and pepper to taste

- 1 lemon, juiced

Preparation:

1. Remove the stiff stems from the collard greens and carefully wash them.

2. Roll the leaves tightly before slicing them into thin ribbons.

3. In a large skillet over medium heat, heat the olive oil.

4. Add minced garlic and red pepper flakes (if using), sauté for 1-2 minutes until fragrant.

5. Add collard greens to the pan, tossing to coat in the garlic-infused oil.

6. Cook for 5-7 minutes until the greens are tender but still vibrant.
7. Season with salt and pepper to taste.
8. Squeeze fresh lemon juice over the collard greens before serving.

Nutritional Value (per serving):

- Calories: Approximately 80
- Protein: 3g
- Fiber: 5g
- Vitamin A: 160% DV
- Vitamin C: 80% DV
- Calcium: 15% DV
- Iron: 2% DV

Enjoy your nutritious and delicious green collard bliss!

10. Cabbage Lime Sensation

Ingredients:

- medium-sized green cabbage, shredded

- limes, juiced

- 1 tablespoon olive oil

- 1 teaspoon honey

- Salt and pepper to taste

- Optional: chopped fresh herbs for garnish

Preparation:

- Combine shredded cabbage in a large mixing dish.

- In a separate bowl, whisk together lime juice, olive oil, honey, salt, and pepper to create the dressing.

- Pour the dressing over the shredded cabbage and toss well to ensure even coating.

- Let the salad marinate for at least 15 minutes to allow flavors to meld.

- If preferred, garnish with fresh herbs before serving.

Nutritional Value (per serving):

- Calories: Approximately 120 kcal

- Protein: 2g

- Fat: 7g

- Carbohydrates: 15g

- Fiber: 6g

- Vitamin C: 80mg (133% DV)

- Calcium: 80mg (8% DV) Iron: 1.5mg (8% DV)

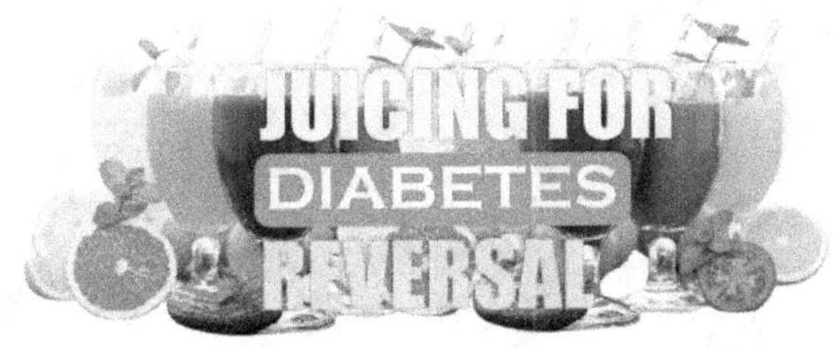

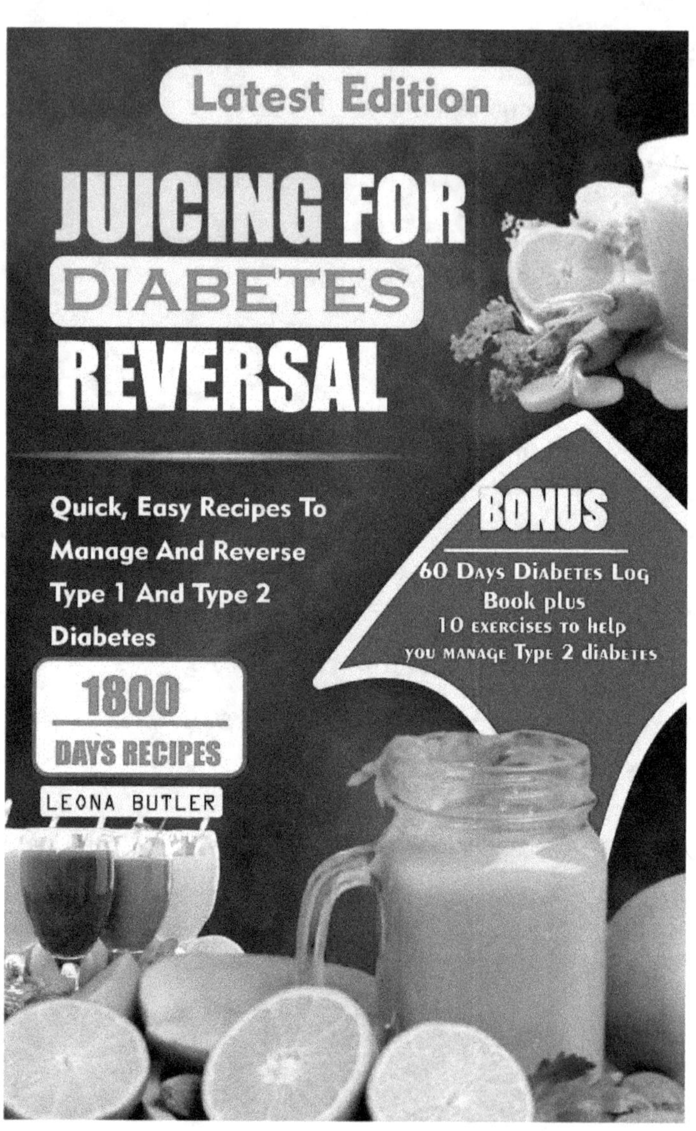

Latest Edition
JUICING FOR DIABETES REVERSAL
Quick, Easy Recipes To Manage And Reverse Type 1 And Type 2 Diabetes
1800 DAYS RECIPES
LEONA BUTLER
BONUS
60 Days Diabetes Log Book plus 10 exercises to help you manage Type 2 diabetes

2. fruit juice recipe for Diabetes reversal

1. Green Goodness Juice:

Ingredients:

- 2 cups spinach leaves
- 1 cucumber, peeled and chopped
- 1 green apple, cored and sliced
- 1 celery stalk, chopped
- 1 lemon, juiced
- 1 inch ginger, peeled
- 1 cup pineapple chunks 1 cup water or coconut water

Preparation:

1. Wash all the vegetables and fruits thoroughly.
2. In a blender, combine spinach, cucumber, green apple, celery, lemon juice, ginger, and pineapple.
3. To achieve the correct consistency, add water or coconut water.
4. Blend until completely smooth.
5. If preferred, strain the juice through a fine mesh sieve or cheesecloth to remove the pulp.
6. Pour into glasses and serve immediately.

Nutritional Value (Approximate):

- Calories: 120

- Total Fat: 0.5g

- Cholesterol: 0mg

- Sodium: 50mg

- Total Carbohydrates: 30g

- Dietary Fiber: 5g

- Sugars: 20g Protein: 3g

2. Berry Bliss Juice

Ingredients:

- 1 cup mixed berries (strawberries, blueberries, raspberries)

- 1 medium-sized banana

- 1/2 cup Greek yogurt

- 1/2 cup almond milk

- 1 tablespoon honey Ice cubes (optional)

Preparation:

1. Wash the berries thoroughly.

2. Peel and slice the banana.

3. In a blender, combine the mixed berries, banana slices, Greek yogurt, almond milk, and honey.

4. Blend until smooth and creamy.

5. If desired, add ice cubes and blend again for a chilled consistency.

6. Pour the Berry Bliss Juice into glasses and serve immediately.

Nutritional Value (approximate per serving):

- Calories: 200

- Protein: 7g

- Fat: 4g

- Carbohydrates: 40g

- Fiber: 5g

- Sugars: 28g

- Vitamin C: 45mg

- Calcium: 150mg

3. Citrus Delight Juice: Citrus Delight Juice:

Ingredients:

- 2 large oranges, peeled and segmented
- grapefruit, peeled and segmented
- lemons, juiced
- 1 tablespoon honey 1 cup cold water Ice cubes (optional)

Preparation:

1. Combine the orange segments, grapefruit segments, and lemon juice in a blender.
2. Add honey and cold water to the blender.
3. Blend until smooth.
4. If preferred, strain the mixture to eliminate any pulp.
5. Serve over ice cubes if you prefer a chilled drink.

Nutritional Value (per serving):

- Calories: 120
- Total Fat: 0g
- Cholesterol: 0mg
- Sodium: 5mg
- Total Carbohydrates: 31g

- Dietary Fiber: 4g

- Sugars: 22g

- Protein: 2g

4. Carrot Zinger Juice

Ingredients:

- 4 large carrots, washed and peeled

- 1 medium-sized ginger root, peeled

- 1 lemon, peeled and segmented 1 medium-sized apple, cored and sliced

Preparation:

1. Cut the carrots, ginger, lemon segments, and apple slices into sizes suitable for your juicer.
2. Feed the ingredients into the juicer one by one.
3. Once all ingredients are juiced, stir the mixture well.
4. Pour the juice into the glasses and serve right away.

Nutritional Value (per serving):

- Calories: approximately 120
- Carbohydrates: 30g
- Dietary Fiber: 6g
- Sugars: 18g
- Vitamin A: 240% DV
- Vitamin C: 70% DV
- Iron: 2% DV

5. Green apple delight juice

Ingredients:

- 4 medium-sized green apples, cored and sliced
- 1 cucumber, peeled and chopped
- 1 celery stalk, chopped
- 1 cup fresh spinach leaves
- 1 lemon, juiced
- tablespoon ginger, grated
- 1-2 cups cold water or ice cubes (adjust for desired consistency)

Preparation:

1. Place sliced green apples, cucumber, celery, spinach, lemon juice, and grated ginger in a blender.
2. Add cold water or ice cubes to achieve your preferred thickness.
3. Blend until smooth.
4. Strain the juice using a fine mesh sieve or cheesecloth to remove pulp, if desired. Pour the juice into glasses and serve chilled.

6. Pineapple Mint Refresher

Ingredients:

- cups fresh pineapple chunks
- 1/4 cup fresh mint leaves
- 1 tablespoon honey or agave syrup
- 1 cup ice cubes
- 1 cup cold water

Optional:

Mint sprigs and pineapple slices for garnish

Preparation:

1. In a blender, combine the fresh pineapple chunks, mint leaves, honey (or agave syrup), and ice cubes.

2. Add cold water to the blender.

3. Combine the ingredients in a blender until smooth and well blended.

4. Taste and adjust sweetness if needed by adding more honey or agave syrup.

5. Pour the mixture into glasses over ice.

6. Garnish with mint sprigs and pineapple slices if desired.

7. Turmeric Twist Juice:

Ingredients:

- 2 large oranges, peeled and segmented
- 1 medium-sized carrot, peeled and chopped
- 1 inch fresh turmeric root, peeled and sliced
- 1/2 inch ginger root, peeled and sliced
- 1 small apple, cored and chopped
- 1 cup cold water Ice cubes (optional)

Preparation:

1. Place the oranges, carrot, turmeric, ginger, and apple in a blender.
2. Add cold water and blend until smooth.
3. To remove the pulp, strain the juice through a fine mesh screen or cheesecloth.
4. Pour the juice into glasses over ice cubes if desired.

Nutritional Value (per serving):

- Calories: 120
- Total Fat: 0.5g
- Cholesterol: 0mg
- Sodium: 10mg
- Total Carbohydrates: 30g
- Dietary Fiber: 5g
- Sugars: 20g
- Protein: 2g
- Vitamin C: 90% DV
- Vitamin A: 120% DV
- Iron: 4% DV

8. Cucumber Lime Cooler

Ingredients:

- large cucumber, peeled and sliced

- limes, juiced

- 2 tablespoons honey

- 1 cup ice cubes

- 1 cup cold water

- Fresh mint leaves for garnish

Preparation:

1. In a blender, combine the peeled and sliced cucumber, lime juice, honey, ice cubes, and cold water.

2. Blend until smooth and well combined.

3. Strain the mixture using a fine-mesh sieve to remove any pulp, if desired.

4. Pour the refreshing cooler into glasses over ice.

5. Garnish with fresh mint leaves. Stir well before serving.

Ingredients:

- 4 cups diced watermelon
- 1/4 cup fresh basil leaves
- 1 tablespoon honey
- lime, juiced
- cups cold water
- Ice cubes

Preparation:

1. In a blender, combine diced watermelon, fresh basil leaves, honey, and lime juice.
2. Blend until smooth.
3. If preferred, strain the mixture to eliminate any pulp.In a large pitcher, mix the watermelon-basil blend with cold water.
4. Refrigerate for at least 1 hour. Serve over ice cubes.

10. Pear - flection juice

Ingredients:

- 4 ripe pears, peeled and chopped
- 1 cup water
- tablespoon lemon juice
- teaspoons honey (adjust to taste) Ice cubes (optional)

Preparation:

1. In a blender, combine chopped pears, water, lemon juice, and honey. Blend until smooth and well combined.
2. Strain the mixture using a fine mesh sieve to remove pulp, if desired.
3. Allow at least 30 minutes before serving to chill. Serve over ice cubes if preferred.

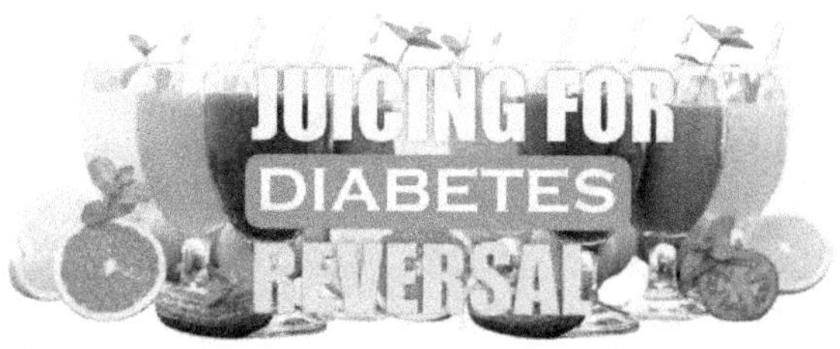

3. Vegetable juice recipe for Diabetes reversal

1.Green Machine Delight:

Ingredients:

- 2 cups fresh spinach leaves

- 1 cup kale, chopped

- 1 medium cucumber, peeled and sliced

- 1 green apple, cored and diced

- 1/2 lemon, juiced

- 1 tablespoon chia seeds

- 1 cup coconut water Ice cubes (optional)

Preparation:

1. Wash the spinach and kale thoroughly.

2. In a blender, combine spinach, kale, cucumber, green apple, and chia seeds.

3. Fill the mixer halfway with lemon juice.

4. Pour in coconut water.

5. Blend until smooth. Add ice cubes if desired for a colder drink.

6. Pour into a glass and enjoy your nutrient-packed Green Machine Delight!

Ingredients:

- 2 medium-sized cucumbers
- 1/2 red onion, finely diced
- 1/2 cup cherry tomatoes, halved
- 1/4 cup feta cheese, crumbled
- 2 tablespoons olive oil
- 1 tablespoon balsamic vinegar
- 1 teaspoon honey
- Freshly ground black pepper to taste
- 1 tablespoon chopped
  fresh mint or parsley for
  garnish

Preparation:

1. Peel and dice the cucumbers into bite-sized pieces.
2. In a bowl, combine diced cucumbers, finely diced red onion, halved cherry tomatoes, and crumbled feta cheese.
3. In a separate small bowl, whisk together olive oil, balsamic vinegar, honey, and black pepper to make the dressing.
4. Toss the cucumber mixture slightly with the dressing to coat.
5. Let the salad marinate in the refrigerator for at least 30 minutes to enhance flavors. Before

serving, garnish with chopped fresh mint or parsley.

3. Turmeric Tonic

Ingredients:

- 1 cup water

- 1 teaspoon turmeric powder

- 1 tablespoon honey

- 1 tablespoon freshly squeezed lemon juice

- A pinch of black pepper

Preparation

1. Heat 1 cup of water in a saucepan.

2. Add 1 teaspoon of turmeric powder to the hot water and stir well.

3. Allow the mixture to simmer for 5 minutes, ensuring the turmeric is fully dissolved.

4. Remove from heat and let it cool for a minute.

5. Stir in 1 tablespoon each of honey and freshly squeezed lemon juice.

6. Add a pinch of black pepper and mix thoroughly.

7. Strain the tonic to remove any sediment.

8. Pour the turmeric tonic into a cup and enjoy!

4. Leafy Greens Elixir

Ingredients:

- 2 cups fresh spinach leaves

- 1 cup kale, chopped

- 1 cucumber, peeled and sliced

- 1 green apple, cored and diced

- 1 lemon, juiced

- 1-inch piece of ginger, peeled

- 1 cup water or coconut water Ice cubes (optional)

Preparation:

1. Wash the spinach and kale thoroughly.

2. In a blender, combine spinach, kale, cucumber, green apple, lemon juice, and ginger.

3. To achieve the correct consistency, add water or coconut water.

4. Blend until smooth.

5. Strain the mixture if a smoother texture is preferred.

6. Serve over ice cubes if desired.

Nutritional Value (per serving):

- Calories: 90

- Protein: 3g

- Fiber: 5g

- Vitamin A: 160% DV

- Vitamin C: 120% DV

- Iron: 10% DV

- Calcium: 8% DV

Enjoy this nutrient-packed leafy greens elixir for a refreshing and healthy boost!

5. Beet Bliss Blend

Ingredients:

- 2 medium-sized beets, peeled and chopped

- 1 cup fresh strawberries, hulled

- 1 ripe banana

- 1/2 cup Greek yogurt

- 1 tablespoon chia seeds

- 1 cup almond milk

- 1 teaspoon honey (optional) Ice cubes (optional)

Preparation:

1. Place chopped beets, strawberries, banana, Greek yogurt, chia seeds, and almond milk in a blender.
2. Blend until smooth and creamy.
3. Add honey if desired for sweetness.
4. If a colder consistency is preferred, add ice cubes and blend again.
5. Pour into glasses and serve immediately.

Nutritional Value (per serving):

- Calories: 180
- Protein: 8g
- Carbohydrates: 32g
- Fiber: 7g Fat: 3.5g
- Vitamins and minerals: Rich in Vitamin C, potassium, and antioxidants.

6. Tomato Basil Refresher

Ingredients:

- 4 large tomatoes, diced

- 1 cup fresh basil leaves

- cucumber, peeled and diced

- 1/2 red onion, finely chopped

- cloves garlic, minced 3 cups vegetable broth

- 1/4 cup balsamic vinegar

- Salt and pepper to taste

- Ice cubes (optional)

Preparation:

1. In a blender, combine diced tomatoes, basil leaves, cucumber, red onion, and minced garlic.

2. Blend until smooth, gradually adding vegetable broth and balsamic vinegar.

3. Season with salt and pepper to taste, blending again to incorporate.

4. Strain the mixture to remove any pulp if desired.

5. Before serving, chill the soup for at least 2 hours. Serve chilled, optionally over ice cubes.

7. Fiber-Rich Fusion

Ingredients:

- 2 cups mixed salad greens (spinach, kale, arugula)
- 1 cup quinoa, cooked
- 1 cup chickpeas, drained and rinsed
- 1 cup cherry tomatoes, halved
- 1 cucumber, diced
- avocado, sliced
- 1/4 cup pumpkin seeds
- tablespoons olive oil
- 1 tablespoon balsamic vinegar Salt and pepper to taste

Preparation:

1. In a large bowl, combine the mixed salad greens, cooked quinoa, chickpeas, cherry tomatoes, cucumber, avocado, and pumpkin seeds.
2. In a small bowl, whisk together the olive oil, balsamic vinegar, salt, and pepper to create the dressing.
3. Drizzle the dressing over the salad and gently toss to coat all of the ingredients.
4. Serve immediately, enjoying a fiber-packed and nutrient-rich fusion salad.

Nutritional Value (per serving):

- Calories: 400

- Protein: 12g

- Carbohydrates: 45g

- Fiber: 10g

- Fat: 20g

This Fiber-Rich Fusion Salad provides a wholesome mix of vitamins, minerals, and dietary fiber, making it a delicious and nutritious option for a balanced meal.

8. Gingered Carrot Crush

Ingredients:

- 4 cups carrots, peeled and grated

- tablespoon fresh ginger, grated

- tablespoons olive oil

- 1 tablespoon honey

- 1 tablespoon lemon juice

- Salt and pepper to taste

- Optional: chopped fresh herbs for garnish

Preparation:

1. Warm the olive oil in a large skillet over medium heat.

2. Add grated carrots and sauté for 5-7 minutes until they begin to soften.

3. Stir in fresh ginger and continue to cook for an additional 2-3 minutes.

4. Drizzle honey and lemon juice over the carrot-ginger mixture, stirring well to coat evenly.

5. Season with salt and pepper to taste.

6. Cook for an additional 3-5 minutes until the carrots are tender but still slightly crisp. Remove from heat and garnish with chopped fresh herbs if desired.

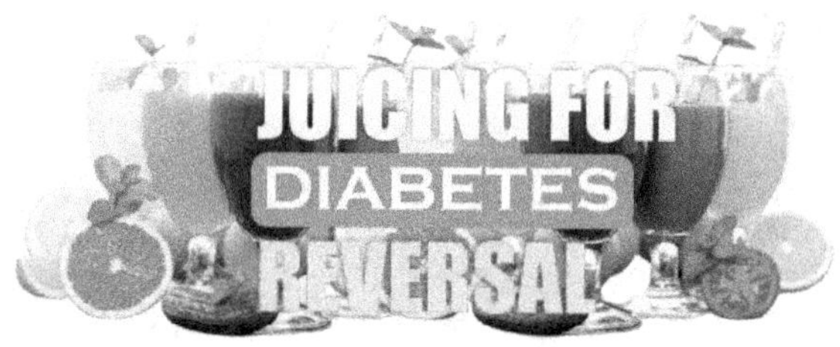

9. Spinach Citrus Symphony

Ingredients:

- 4 cups fresh spinach leaves

- 1 cup orange segments

- 1/2 cup sliced strawberries

- 1/4 cup crumbled feta cheese 1/4 cup chopped walnuts

Citrus Dressing:

- 3 tablespoons olive oil

- 2 tablespoons fresh orange juice

- 1 tablespoon balsamic vinegar

- 1 teaspoon honey

- Salt and pepper to taste

Prepare Salad Base:

- Wash and dry the spinach leaves.

- In a large bowl, combine the spinach, orange segments, sliced strawberries, feta cheese, and chopped walnuts.

Make Citrus Dressing:

- In a small bowl, whisk together olive oil, fresh orange juice, balsamic vinegar, honey, salt, and pepper.

Combine and Toss:

- Pour the citrus dressing over the salad ingredients.
- Gently toss the salad until all ingredients are evenly coated with the dressing.

Serve:

- Divide the salad into individual servings.
- Garnish with more walnuts and feta cheese, if desired.

Nutritional Value (per serving):

- Calories: 250
- Protein: 6g
- Fat: 20g
- Carbohydrates: 15g
- Fiber: 4g
- Vitamin C: 45mg
- Calcium: 120mg

Enjoy this nutritious Spinach Citrus Symphony!

Ingredients

- 2 cups fresh kale, chopped
- 1 cup carrots, julienned
- 1 tablespoon olive oil
- 1 clove garlic, minced
- 1/2 teaspoon salt
- 1/4 teaspoon black pepper
- 1/2 teaspoon lemon juice

Preparation:

1. In a skillet over medium heat, heat the olive oil.

2. Sauté the minced garlic for 1-2 minutes, or until fragrant.

3. Add julienned carrots and cook for 3-4 minutes until slightly softened.

4. Add chopped kale, salt, and black pepper. Stir and cook for an additional 4-5 minutes until kale is tender but still vibrant.

5. Finish with a splash of lemon juice for a burst of freshness. Serve hot as a nutritious side dish.

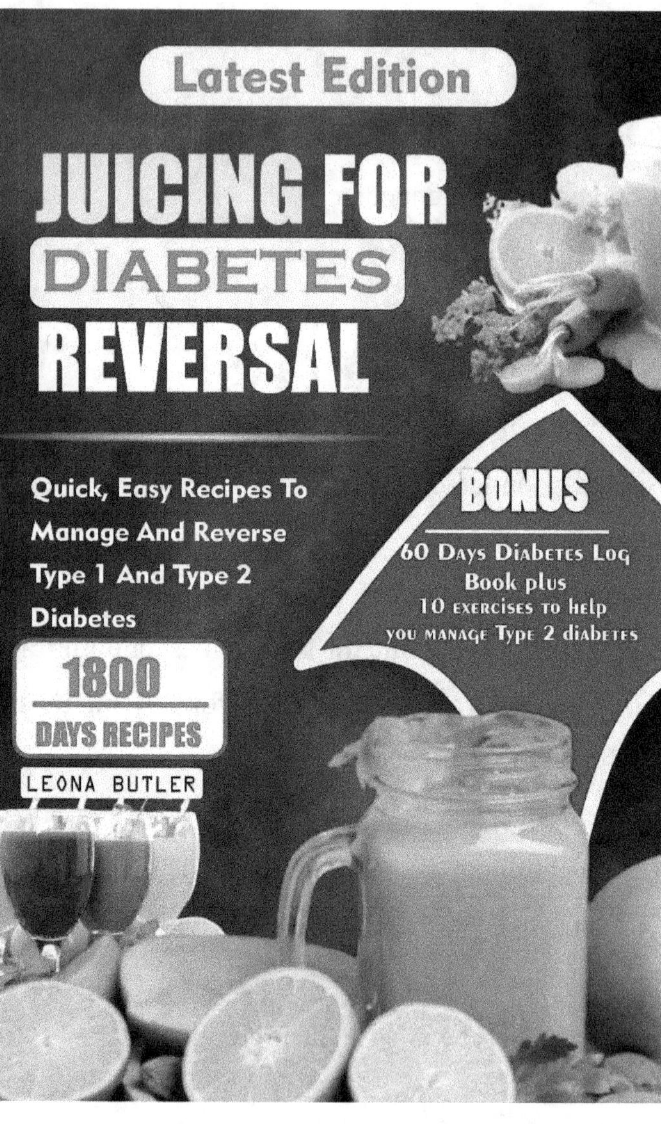

Latest Edition
JUICING FOR DIABETES REVERSAL
Quick, Easy Recipes To Manage And Reverse Type 1 And Type 2 Diabetes
1800 DAYS RECIPES
LEONA BUTLER
BONUS
60 Days Diabetes Log Book plus 10 exercises to help you manage Type 2 diabetes

10 exercises to help you manage Type 2 diabetes

1. Strolling

Walking is a popular low-impact activity that has a plethora of health benefits. It is especially good for diabetics, as it lowers blood pressure, glucose levels, and cholesterol levels. The American Diabetes Association (ADA) recommends 30 minutes of brisk walking each day, which equates to around 100 steps per minute.

Incorporating activities such as stair climbing can help to increase the effectiveness of walks. Those who were not physically active prior to a diabetes diagnosis should begin walking routines slowly and gradually increase the pace. This method allows the body to adjust to greater activity levels without undue stress.

Walking has significant cardiovascular benefits that contribute to general well-being and diabetes management. Regular walking routines are essential for maintaining a healthy lifestyle, aiding in weight management, and lowering the risk of diabetes problems. Walking as a regular exercise, adapted to individual fitness levels, thus seems to be a helpful technique in boosting physical health and efficiently treating diabetes.

2. Jogging

Running, when combined with sufficient training and approval from your healthcare physician, allows you to advance from brisk walking to a more intense activity. This transition has health benefits, including a lower risk of high blood pressure, higher blood sugar levels, and increased cholesterol.

According to the proposal, a moderate approach to running, possibly beginning with brisk walking, can be a positive step toward improving cardiovascular health. It does, however, underline the significance of checking with a healthcare practitioner to ensure that such physical exercise is suitable depending on specific health concerns.

This data emphasizes the potential benefits of adopting running into one's fitness routine, implying a link between this higher-intensity exercise and a reduction in the risk factors connected with cardiovascular disease. It emphasizes the importance of a balanced and gradual training strategy, as well as the requirement for medical supervision to adjust the exercise plan to particular health concerns.

3. Biking

Cycling on a regular basis, whether outdoors on an old cycle or indoors on a stationary bike, has numerous health benefits. Cycling is popular for its benefits to heart and lung health, but it also improves balance and posture. It is not required to purchase an expensive exercise bike; for outdoor rides, an old bike or a stationary bike at a local gym would suffice.

Importantly, research suggests that cycling can help people with diabetes live healthier lives. Cycling's accessibility makes it an appealing fitness alternative, encouraging physical well-being and appealing to a diverse variety of people, from outdoor enthusiasts to gym-goers. Cycling appears as a diverse and useful sport for general health, whether it's the ease of a stationary bike or the delight of bicycling through outdoor landscapes.

4. Dancing

Dancing is a dynamic and pleasurable addition to your training regimen that provides both pleasure and a variety of health benefits. It is known as a heart-healthy activity that can improve fitness and blood sugar control in people with Type 2 Diabetes (T2D). A study found that those with T2D who participated in a dance program were more motivated to stick to a regimen than those who participated in a different fitness program.

The findings highlight the good influence of dance on both the physical and motivational elements of diabetes management.

This type of exercise benefits cardiovascular health, which is critical for those with T2D. Dancing's rhythmic movements encourage greater blood circulation and can help regulate blood sugar levels. Furthermore, the enjoyment associated with dancing can help individuals maintain a consistent exercise schedule, addressing a frequent difficulty in diabetes management—adherence to routine physical activity.

Incorporating dance into one's lifestyle not only adds a fun element to workouts, but it also acts as a holistic approach to improving overall health, making it a helpful option for people looking for effective techniques to manage and improve their well-being while living with diabetes.

5. Aqua aerobics

Water aerobics, particularly swimming, has a variety of benefits, making it an appealing training option. Water's buoyancy reduces joint impact, making it mild on the joints, which is important for those with Type 2 Diabetes (T2D). Furthermore, this type of exercise has the ability to reduce blood sugar levels, aiding with diabetes management.

Swimming, in addition to being beneficial to T2D, improves general fitness by encouraging greater strength and cardiovascular health. Water's resistance forces the engagement of multiple muscle groups, resulting in a full and effective workout. Water aerobics is a wonderful alternative for anyone wishing to maintain or improve their health because of its dual influence on strength and cardiovascular well-being.

In a broader sense, the attraction of water aerobics stems from its accessibility and inclusivity. Because of their low-impact nature, these workouts are appropriate for people of all fitness levels and ages. As a result, water aerobics has emerged as a diverse and helpful exercise technique for not just controlling T2D but also increasing general well-being and fitness.

6. Interval training at high intensity

High-Intensity Interval Training (HIIT) entails alternating between short bursts of high-intensity exercise and longer periods of lower-intensity activity. This adaptable method is applicable to activities such as jogging and cycling. Individuals with Type 2 diabetes, in particular, may benefit from HIIT since exercise has the ability to lower fasting blood sugar levels. The method's efficacy stems from its capacity to improve cardiovascular fitness and metabolic function. It promotes enhanced glucose utilization and insulin sensitivity by pushing the body to its limits during high-intensity periods.

Because of the organized nature of HIIT, quick workouts are possible, making it a time-effective solution for individuals with hectic schedules. This training method's dynamic nature not only benefits in calorie burning but also contributes to post-exercise calorie expenditure, aiding weight management. Incorporating HIIT into a fitness regimen can be good for anyone looking for diverse and impactful workouts while addressing specific health concerns, such as Type 2 diabetes management through blood sugar regulation.

7. Strength training

Weight training is a sort of strength training that uses weights or equipment to increase or maintain muscular growth and strength. It has the potential to improve insulin sensitivity and glucose tolerance in people with Type 2 Diabetes (T2D). This type of physical activity is critical in promoting overall health.

Weight training causes muscle contractions, which leads to muscle development, through systematic resistance workouts. Notably, for those with T2D, increased insulin sensitivity is critical for controlling blood sugar levels. The technique involves muscles using glucose more efficiently, which aids glycemic management. Furthermore, better glucose tolerance is an important result, demonstrating the body's improved ability to handle and process glucose.

Weight training in a fitness routine is beneficial not just for people seeking muscular strength, but also for those dealing with T2D. This type of exercise provides a multimodal approach to diabetes care, addressing both muscle health and metabolic elements, leading to a more comprehensive diabetes control plan. Always contact with a healthcare provider before beginning a new fitness plan, especially if you have a specific health condition like T2D, to ensure safety and effectiveness.

8. Yoga

Yoga, a comprehensive practice that combines low-impact exercise, meditation, and controlled breathing, provides numerous benefits, which are especially beneficial for older people with Type 2 Diabetes (T2D). Yoga's mild nature improves improved balance, flexibility, and strength, addressing concerns about the increased risk of falls among older T2D patients.

Yoga has the ability to manage blood sugar and cholesterol levels in addition to physical benefits. Yoga's thoughtful and contemplative features aid to stress reduction, which is critical for people with T2D who want to control their health.

Yoga activities that emphasize controlled breathing may help improve respiratory function and overall well-being.

Yoga, due to its low-impact nature, is an appropriate workout option for persons with T2D, cultivating a healthy lifestyle without putting undue strain on the body. Incorporating yoga into a practice can contribute to a holistic diabetes care plan, providing both physical and mental well-being advantages.

9. Tai chi

Tai chi is a traditional Chinese martial art that combines low-impact movements, meditation, and concentrated breathing methods. This all-encompassing approach improves balance, range of motion, and overall well-being. The practice's unique combination of physical and mental components makes it an excellent supplement to any training regimen. Notably, the contemplative qualities encourage a sense of calm and mindfulness.

Tai chi's low-impact nature is mild on the joints, making it suitable for people of all fitness levels. Its use in a regular physical routine may have a favorable influence on blood sugar levels. The emphasis on fluid, controlled movements improves flexibility and stability. Furthermore, the meditative component promotes relaxation, which may reduce stress.

Tai chi's historical origins and lasting popularity attest to its effectiveness in fostering physical and mental wellness. It promotes a mind-body connection that goes beyond traditional workout regimens as an integrative discipline. Tai chi's many benefits position it as a comprehensive approach to wellness, embracing physical fitness, mental clarity, and possibly blood sugar regulation.

10. Pilates

Pilates is promoted as a low-impact exercise that emphasizes repetitive motions and breath control in order to improve core strength, balance, and posture. Its placement on this list is justified by the possible benefits it may provide. According to one study, Pilates exercise has been linked to better blood glucose management in those with Type 2 Diabetes (T2D). This type of exercise takes a moderate yet effective approach, making it ideal for anyone looking for a workout that focuses on joint and muscle health.

Pilates motions are repetitious, which helps to strengthen the core muscles, which are important for overall stability. Furthermore, the emphasis on breath control is consistent with the mind-body link, supporting a holistic approach to fitness. The good effect on blood glucose levels adds a valuable dimension, indicating Pilates as a therapeutic practice for those with T2D.

In conclusion, Pilates stands out as a holistic workout program that not only targets core strength, balance, and posture but also has the potential to improve blood glucose control, which is especially important for persons with Type 2 Diabetes.

BONUS: DIABETIC LOG BOOK

THE PAPERBACK OF THIS VERSION HAS A FREE 60 DAYS DIABETIC LOG BOOK

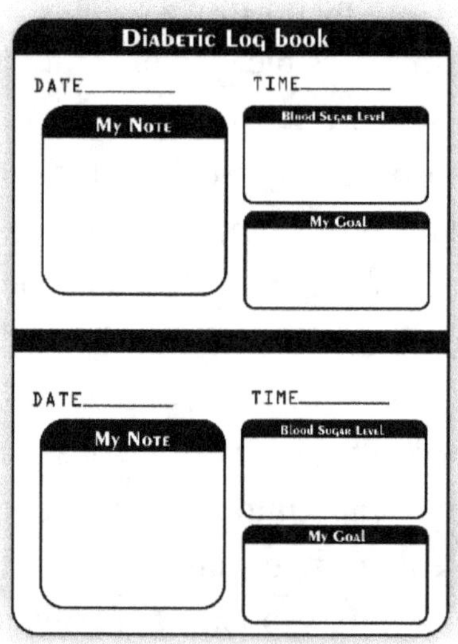

Conclusion

In conclusion, incorporating juicing into a holistic approach to diabetes management has enormous promise for those seeking reversal. The combination of nutrient-rich fruits and vegetables in fresh, homemade juices can help to stabilize blood sugar levels and improve overall health. These drinks' strong antioxidants, vitamins, and minerals not only improve insulin sensitivity but also assist the body's natural healing mechanisms.

It is critical to recognize the synergistic relationship between juicing and lifestyle modifications as we travel the path to diabetes reversal. Adopting a healthy diet, frequent exercise, and stress management in addition to juicing increases the likelihood of favorable outcomes. Furthermore, the individualized nature of juicing allows people to tailor recipes to their specific nutritional needs, providing a long-term and joyful road to better health.

While juicing might be beneficial, it is critical to speak with a healthcare expert for individualized advice and monitoring. Juicing emerges as a tasty ally in the pursuit of diabetes reversal, delivering a refreshing and uplifting avenue towards greater health and vitality when combined with a commitment to wellness and educated choices.

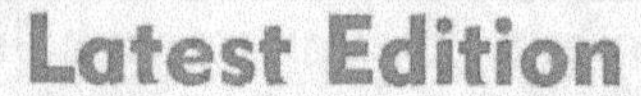

Latest Edition
JUICING FOR DIABETES REVERSAL
Quick, Easy Recipes To Manage And Reverse Type 1 And Type 2 Diabetes
1800 DAYS RECIPES
LEONA BUTLER
BONUS
60 Days Diabetes Log Book plus
10 exercises to help you manage Type 2 diabetes

Diabetic Log book

DATE _______________   **TIME** _______________

My Note

Blood Sugar Level

My Goal

DATE _______________   **TIME** _______________

My Note

Blood Sugar Level

My Goal

Diabetic Log book

DATE__________   TIME__________

My Note

Blood Sugar Level

My Goal

DATE__________   TIME__________

My Note

Blood Sugar Level

My Goal

Diabetic Log book

DATE_____________ TIME_____________

My Note

Blood Sugar Level

My Goal

DATE_____________ TIME_____________

My Note

Blood Sugar Level

My Goal

Diabetic Log book

DATE_______________   **TIME**_______________

My Note

Blood Sugar Level

My Goal

DATE_______________   **TIME**_______________

My Note

Blood Sugar Level

My Goal

Diabetic Log book

DATE________________

TIME________________

My Note

Blood Sugar Level

My Goal

DATE________________

TIME________________

My Note

Blood Sugar Level

My Goal

Diabetic Log book

DATE_________

TIME_________

My Note

Blood Sugar Level

My Goal

DATE_________

TIME_________

My Note

Blood Sugar Level

My Goal

Diabetic Log book

DATE________________   TIME________________

My Note

Blood Sugar Level

My Goal

DATE________________   TIME________________

My Note

Blood Sugar Level

My Goal

Diabetic Log book

DATE________________   TIME________________

My Note

Blood Sugar Level

My Goal

DATE________________   TIME________________

My Note

Blood Sugar Level

My Goal

Diabetic Log book

DATE________________   TIME______________

My Note

Blood Sugar Level

My Goal

DATE________________   TIME______________

My Note

Blood Sugar Level

My Goal

Diabetic Log book

DATE________

TIME________

My Note

Blood Sugar Level

My Goal

DATE________

TIME________

My Note

Blood Sugar Level

My Goal

Diabetic Log book

DATE_________ TIME_________

My Note

Blood Sugar Level

My Goal

DATE_________ TIME_________

My Note

Blood Sugar Level

My Goal

Diabetic Log book

DATE__________   TIME__________

My Note

Blood Sugar Level

My Goal

DATE__________   TIME__________

My Note

Blood Sugar Level

My Goal

Diabetic Log book

DATE________

TIME________

My Note

Blood Sugar Level

My Goal

DATE________

TIME________

My Note

Blood Sugar Level

My Goal

Diabetic Log book

DATE__________   TIME__________

My Note

Blood Sugar Level

My Goal

DATE__________   TIME__________

My Note

Blood Sugar Level

My Goal

Diabetic Log book

DATE_________________

TIME_________________

My Note

Blood Sugar Level

My Goal

DATE_________________

TIME_________________

My Note

Blood Sugar Level

My Goal

Diabetic Log book

DATE_________   TIME_________

My Note

Blood Sugar Level

My Goal

DATE_________   TIME_________

My Note

Blood Sugar Level

My Goal

Diabetic Log book

DATE_____________   TIME_____________

My Note

Blood Sugar Level

My Goal

DATE_____________   TIME_____________

My Note

Blood Sugar Level

My Goal

Diabetic Log book

DATE___________   **TIME**___________

My Note

Blood Sugar Level

My Goal

DATE___________   **TIME**___________

My Note

Blood Sugar Level

My Goal

Diabetic Log book

DATE________________

TIME________________

My Note

Blood Sugar Level

My Goal

DATE________________

TIME________________

My Note

Blood Sugar Level

My Goal

Diabetic Log book

DATE__________

TIME__________

My Note

Blood Sugar Level

My Goal

DATE__________

TIME__________

My Note

Blood Sugar Level

My Goal

Diabetic Log book

DATE_______________   TIME_______________

My Note

Blood Sugar Level

My Goal

DATE_______________   TIME_______________

My Note

Blood Sugar Level

My Goal

Diabetic Log book

DATE______________   TIME______________

My Note

Blood Sugar Level

My Goal

DATE______________   TIME______________

My Note

Blood Sugar Level

My Goal

Diabetic Log book

DATE____________

TIME____________

My Note

Blood Sugar Level

My Goal

DATE____________

TIME____________

My Note

Blood Sugar Level

My Goal

Diabetic Log book

DATE________

TIME________

My Note

Blood Sugar Level

My Goal

DATE________

TIME________

My Note

Blood Sugar Level

My Goal

Diabetic Log book

DATE__________   TIME__________

My Note

Blood Sugar Level

My Goal

DATE__________   TIME__________

My Note

Blood Sugar Level

My Goal

Diabetic Log book

DATE_____________   **TIME**_____________

My Note

Blood Sugar Level

My Goal

DATE_____________   **TIME**_____________

My Note

Blood Sugar Level

My Goal

Diabetic Log book

DATE______________

TIME______________

My Note

Blood Sugar Level

My Goal

DATE______________

TIME______________

My Note

Blood Sugar Level

My Goal

Diabetic Log book

DATE_________________

TIME____________

My Note

Blood Sugar Level

My Goal

DATE_________________

TIME____________

My Note

Blood Sugar Level

My Goal

9 7 9 8 8 7 4 2 0 3 5 3 5